The Devil's Diet

By Anita Lover

Sinuous Publications

ISBN 978-1-4116-9532-0

This book wouldn't have been possible without
dd (the best winker ever),
JB, and Cherry Cherry.

Contents

"I can resist everything except temptation"— Oscar Wilde

Introduction

Let's start with a simple fact:

You don't know how to lose weight.

I know that sounds harsh—very harsh and unpleasant. But why else would you be reading this book? You might even try saying it to yourself for a little reinforcement:

I don't know how to lose weight.

Oh sure, you might have a pretty good idea. You've

probably lost eight or ten pounds at some point in your life (and then quickly gained it back…plus some). You may have read every diet book and you probably own a basement full of exercise gadgets. You may know more about calorie counting, interval training and carb-free food than anyone in your zip code.

But, if you haven't actually lost weight and kept it off, you don't really <u>know</u> how to lose weight. That's the simple fact of the matter. There must be gaps in your knowledge or else you would be at your ideal weight.

That's ok—that's right—it's ok. We're going to work on that. Just like learning to be a lawyer or a doctor, losing weight is a complicated business…you can't learn how to really do it overnight. What you need to absorb for now is that there are some weaknesses in what you know. There are a few things that you just haven't figured out. Some mysteries…

One thing that you'll discover is that it takes time to learn enough about your body and your environment. It takes time to develop the habits that you'll need to change your weight. It takes time to train your body to get enough exercise. It takes time to learn which are the right foods for you and how to control your appetite.

It may even take time to develop the patience to make it all work—we all want to drop that weight in the next day or two…when we want something, we're all used to getting it quickly. We take out a credit card, drive to a mall, and buy it.

Weight loss is different. It's not something that you can work hard at for a day or a week and realistically expect to succeed. Try to think of it this way: it took you years and years to put on that weight. At the very least, it's going to take months to get it off. And actually, that's a big part of losing weight—you need to think in terms of weeks and months and everybody has a tough time understanding things in those terms. It's a long slow process.

Why did I write this book?

I'm 35 pounds lighter than I was at my worst, that's why. As a matter of fact, I've lost that 35 pounds three different times, but now I've finally kept it off for the last four years. So I think I have a pretty good idea on what it really takes to lose weight. Back in 2002, I weighed 35 pounds more than I did this morning. No matter how you look at it, that's a big loss and I'm very glad that I was able to do it. Actually, the word 'glad' doesn't quite cover it. I'm *ecstatic*. I'd been trying—for more than twenty years—to control my weight and had seen it steadily creep up. I've always exercised as hard as I could and I've always been on one diet or another. Even so, at one point, I weighed 40 pounds more than the number on my driver's license.

And the funny thing is that all that time I thought I knew

how to lose weight, but I just couldn't do it. At times, it seemed impossible…maybe there was something wrong with me …maybe there was something different about me…there must be something unfair about my metabolism…does any of that sound familiar? After all, there is only one way to lose weight and we all know the formula:

(1) Eat less, and

(2) Exercise more.

That's what all the doctors tell us and they're a bunch of geniuses. Seems simple, right?

It's not simple at all. In fact, if you've been trying to lose weight for years, you probably get a little angry when someone tells you to eat less and exercise more. Easy enough for them to say, right? There are only two things to remember…the part about eating…and the part about exercising. Only an idiot can't do that. And when you fail, you start to think of yourself as an idiot. This is why you feel a little angry or a little hopeless or a little desperate when some skinny guy appears in public and says, 'Eat less and exercise more'.

However, as in most things in life, it's not quite that simple. In fact, it's incredibly complex when you study this subject in detail. What makes it so complicated? Your body,

4

your emotions, your habits, your job, your friends, your family and everything else. All of that makes it very difficult to exercise enough and to diet enough to really lose that weight.

So the idea is to learn about how all the complexities of your life affect your weight and how to overcome those obstacles. Basically, you'll identify what works, what doesn't, and then you'll apply that knowledge.

This is not quick.

This is not easy (nor is it exceptionally difficult).

But anything worth doing is worth taking the time to do it right. Luckily, you have the rest of your life to figure this out. That's right, you're used to thinking in terms of the last 24 hours and how you've failed your diet once again. But that's nothing…chances are you have years and years in front of you to figure all this out. The last 24 hours might have been just one more lesson in what not to do. Did you starve yourself all day before gobbling down an extra-large butterscotch sundae at the ice cream parlor? Well, perhaps the part of the day you starved yourself was part of the problem. Perhaps you need to pace yourself in order to control that binging that happens every so often. It's not easy to learn what pace works for you, but you have decades to figure it out. So let's get started…

So—what about the **sin** part of this book? That might be

why you bought this book and there hasn't been a word about it yet. Well, that's coming next. I'll get to my secrets about how to diet and exercise later. The first thing I'm going to cover is sin. And after that, you'll be anxious to learn everything I can tell you about diet and exercise. All else follows from sin...

1. Sinful Motivations

A sin is a "transgression from the law of God". This is serious stuff for many people and you might want to stop right here if you're a devout Christian or a committed follower of almost any other religion. And if that stops you—that's fine—but please note: you're going to need to find another source for your motivation.

And it had better be a good one because what you're using now isn't working.

So, let's get to it…which of the Ten Commandments are

we going to violate? Patience, keep reading…

This chapter covers different aspects of this delightfully wicked way to motivate yourself. This is so you will understand in depth and in detail why this is important. There are three sections in this chapter which cover the three most important questions: (1) Why is motivation so important? (2) As if you haven't guessed yet…what exactly is this motivation? (3) Why don't more people do this?

So on to the first question…

Why is motivation so important?

The importance of finding a strong motivation to lose weight *cannot be over-emphasized*. Think about it…most people want to lose weight because they want to look better or they want to be healthier or both. At first glance, these seem to be very powerful incentives. Almost everybody understands that fat people are less attractive, and they might even realize that all that fat will eventually kill them.

Yet, they still can't get it done.

You'd think that becoming more attractive is a powerful motivation. Everybody likes attention from the opposite sex and, according to statistics, attractive people make more money and live more contented lives. Certainly, the risk of death should be enough to fill the health clubs. If there's anything that everybody is afraid of, it's death,

However, it's too easy to convince yourself that you still look good with that extra 20 pounds around your middle and that nobody really notices that your jaw line has disappeared into a chubby chinstrap. Many people convince themselves that they're getting enough exercise to be one of those 'fit and fat' people who will outlive all the skinny people because *they're* the ones who are *really* in shape. All-righty then. That's exactly how it works with most people and this is a big reason why many diets don't work.

So they think they're still attractive. And they think they're still healthy.

Let's be very clear about what that exactly means: these are <u>delusions</u>.

Delusions…that's a strong word and I hope that it doesn't offend anybody, but the facts are undeniable. Statistically, overweight people are seen as less attractive and they will die sooner. Period, end of discussion. So if you're overweight and have convinced yourself that you are somewhat attractive and perfectly healthy, chances are that you are operating under a delusion. It's a very common delusion, but it's still a delusion. And it's time to try to see past it.

Here's a little test: find someone thin and then compare them to *anyone* of the same age who is overweight or obese…for most people, it's not even close. Being thin is *the* biggest factor in how attractive you appear to the opposite sex. And the strangest thing about this is that even the heaviest people think that the slim people are more attractive. There's something very ironic about that, but anyway…

Since most people understand the consequences, then why are there so many overweight people? It's simple: these motivations don't work for most people. It's amazing, but the facts speak for themselves. Most people understand the consequences of being overweight, yet the vast majority of people cannot lose any weight.

Let's face it. If you're aware of the health issues and you don't like what you see in the mirror any more—yet you still haven't lost weight…it's time to find something new.

What is the motivation?

So—whatever we use, we know that we're going to need some much **stronger** than mere statistics and fuzzy notions about who is more attractive. We need something all-powerful. Something that goes to the core of our animal being. After all, we're fighting the primitive urge to eat to stay alive. It's hard to do that with just the conscious part of your brain. The good news is that there is a drive that can trump the subtle and persistent compulsion to eat: It is Sex. You might laugh...Sex? Then you might say, I get laid about five times a year and it isn't even that good. How is that supposed to keep me motivated? Well, that's not the kind of sex that we're going to be talking about...

Commandment Number Seven from the Bible states that, you "shall not commit adultery". Commandment Number Ten states that you "shall not covet your neighbor's wife". I suspect, to be fair, that Commandment Number Ten also covers coveting your neighbor's husband.

Have you guessed where you're going to find your motivation now? For those of us in committed relationships, we're going back on the hunt. That's right. As of right now, *you're back in the game*. Get used to it.

Welcome back.

Let's get to work.

Do you remember how you used to think and feel back in high school? Do you remember the thrill the first time a boy asked you to a dance? Do you remember your first French kiss? That little warm twinge has faded, right? As the song says, the thrill is gone. You might not even remember what it feels like. It's been years—you've grown used to your partner and your partner has grown used to you. And you both take each other for granted.

Well, you might say, it's not that bad. You each know how to get the other off. There's a certain formula there and a certain reliability. You don't need to worry about diseases as you did when you were single. Okay, maybe it's not happening as often as you'd like. And maybe the orgasms are less like a stick of dynamite and more like a damp firecracker. Do you still give and get oral sex? Do you look at each other during oral sex or is there a big belly blocking the view? I know, that's a very rough thing to point out. But sometimes I wonder if that post-honeymoon 50 pounds says more about how much love there really is than all the flowery words in the yearly Valentine. If you really loved your partner, shouldn't you *want* to stay attractive? Shouldn't you find a *way* to keep that weight off?

This discussion could get much darker, so I'll stop myself here. Admittedly, this is not a very positive train of thought, but I've ridden this train for too long and I'm sure that some of you have had similar thoughts or worse.

What should be clear is that sex for many of us isn't what it once was—it's not even close. Sure, there aren't gallons of hormones pumping though your veins like when you were a teenager, but should it be this bad? I remember not so long ago when just about everyone in the opposite sex looked hot. About 50% were on my 'to-do' list and many of the others were there after a few glasses of wine. But then, a few years rolled by and they didn't look so good. Even the movie stars started looking flawed. That one has a big nose, that one is too skinny, and that one has a chicken neck. I had never noticed all those lines on their foreheads and those bags under their eyes. Was I turning gay?

No. It has all changed for me and it can change for you too. At least from my experience, all of that can be changed by thinking about—and, perhaps, actively pursuing—adulterous liaisons.

However, you might say, it's not that easy. I can't just cruise around town and start going wild. This is very complicated stuff and there's quite a bit at stake. That's true. There are many different reasons why people don't do this—that's why it seems so complicated—but instead of just giving up, let's take a hard look at the usual reasons and maybe it won't look so bad. If fact, I think that you'll find that some of the reasons are valid and that some of the reasons are imaginary. And then we just need to think about what the real problems might be and how you might solve those problems.

Why don't more people do this?

When you look at it carefully, marriage is a strange concept.

13

Sure, it's great that two people take care of each other and grow old together, sharing their memories and everything...all of that still makes sense to me. Yet there are many people who love sex and love sex with new partners most of all. So why aren't love affairs more common?

It's all the other stuff that gets involved. There are all sorts of unwritten rules and many of these unwritten rules are there to get in the way. I suspect that some of these rules are there to slow down the teenagers and that's probably a good thing. To be 16 and pregnant is not a good path to be on. Most reasonable people would agree that it's smart to slow down the 'sexual debut' of kids until they're a little older and a little wiser. However, after you have a few years behind you and you understand everything that is involved in a sexual relationship, there's really no reason for letting these unwritten rules affect you any more. They're nothing more than childish notions.

Here's one example of an unwritten rule: a married woman shouldn't be associating frequently with men who are not her husband. How strange is that! If you're heterosexual, by definition you are attracted to the opposite sex...and then you're supposed to avoid them? This is very unnatural and such a shame. We all know that these types of friendships can be wonderful—especially when there is a naughty little undercurrent of sexual tension.

With time, there are some women who take this unwritten rule to heart and they begin to regard men with coldness or even hostility. They think that every man is only out to put another notch on his gun (so to speak) and the last thing they want to be is the latest conquest of someone who fancies himself as a stud. Conquests? I think that word disguises another unwritten rule. I've never really understood how someone is 'conquered' like this. Is this really a war? Have we somehow turned sex into a fight? When you stop and think about it, a word like 'conquest' is designed to bring up all sorts of negative emotions about having sex. Yet, there doesn't seem to be any connection to the real meaning of the word.

Another unwritten rule (and perhaps related to the notion of 'conquests') is that sex is a winner-take-all game. It's a competition and we all want to beat out the rest of the world. Then, once you're married, the game is over. You are the champion and it's time to pack on a few dozen pounds. You've come in first and everyone else has come in last.

It's not very hard to find proof that people treat sex like a game. Have you ever seen how competitive people become on TV dating shows? When you sit back and look at those things from a different perspective, it's absolutely crazy to see how so competitive those people can get. It happens all the time. They line up a bunch of gorgeous women who compete for a guy who they wouldn't even bother talking to in real life. Their competitive instincts and their egos take over until pretty soon they're doing all sorts of foolish things. It sounds pretty stupid when you look at it like that.

To me, it seems like a very healthy first step to force yourself to stop thinking about sex as a competition…which leaves me with a bit of a problem. What is it really? Is it a pastime or what? Well, maybe…but one thing is for sure: I have a helluva hobby.

In my weaker moments, when the notion that it is a competition comes back to me (maybe it's just too ingrained), I can still manage. If it is a competition, what does it matter if I don't come in first? I'm more than happy when I finish second or third—I've still beaten everyone else. And the trophies are just as good, if not better. Tee-hee.

So just relax and don't worry about things so much. Do you really care any more if your spouse is having a fling? There was a day when that idea would have made me crazy. I had 'won' the game and how dare someone else start playing with my prize. But now, as long as I don't actually have to witness anything (and it doesn't affect my health), I'm not sure that I care all that much if my spouse is getting a little on the side. After all, is it really such a big deal or are you just getting upset about an unwritten rule that was written by adolescents? And there are more of these childish ideas out there…

Here's another unwritten rule: the worst thing in the world is to be a liar and an adulterer is the biggest liar of them all. If you're like most people, you were probably married in a church and even people who aren't very religious seem to want you to stick to every syllable of the marriage vow that you made before God. Or at least, they want you to stick to the part of the marriage vows that everybody seems to emphasize. You're not supposed to be in the least bit unfaithful. But is it that simple?

But what about the vow to love and respect? Wasn't that in the vows too? Isn't 'love and respect' supposed to work both ways? Do you really think that you are being loved and respected? Did that include your partner gaining 50 pounds? Could gaining all that weight be just as bad as being unfaithful? Okay, maybe what I'm suggesting is a bit of a double standard, but what's important here is that, to many people, love and respect is reflected in a million different things. How do you treat each other? Do you still try to make yourself attractive? Are you really working as hard as you can on *everything*? In my opinion, the 'love and respect' is a black and white issue. There are no shades of gray here. You are either doing everything that you're capable of to show your love and respect, or you're not. Whitening your teeth and paying attention to your hair is great, but it's a waste of everybody's time if you're wearing filthy clothes. Or if you're obese. Love and respect: it's either there or it's not. And, honestly, it's just too difficult for far too many couples. Very few people can actually live up to those standards. It's sad, but nevertheless, the fact is that many couples have already broken their vows.

Perhaps, to take this a step further, it's the *ultimate* disrespect to let yourself go. Is that really the same person I married so many years ago? Did I did agree to spend the rest of my life with a soft sickly thing with a beach ball beer belly? Have I been lied to every day of our marriage?

But (they will say) you fell in love with and married the person who happens to be inside that body…oh, but wait—that's the same person who didn't warn me about what might happen. The same person who stopped trying. There really is no defense.

But I know—there's much more to this. We've talked about a few unwritten rules and what people expect out of marriage vows. It's not easy, is it? This is a *very* complex subject and we need to think through all the angles. So what if marriage isn't perfect—what is? We also need to talk about some of the potential problems with fooling around. If we're going to get serious about this, *let's get serious* and talk about some things that you should be worried about.

We can't live in a fantasy world. There are some very

real problems that can occur with adulterous relationships and we need to address them.

First of all—let's face it, <u>adultery</u> is a loaded word, a very loaded word. The word itself sounds so ugly, and, true, there are very good reasons why it disgusts many people. It reeks of home-wreckers and STDs and hookers—it's a spoiler of lives and health. And it was probably a very good thing for society that it was written into religious law as a mortal sin. If there hadn't been any good controls on adultery, then there would have been huge problems. Throughout history there has been pressure against it and severe consequences for those who get caught.

But things are now a-changing.

The first and foremost question on most minds is this: what might be said about me if someone found out? The vast majority of people frown on this type of behavior. For every open-minded soul, there are a thousand bitches and bastards waiting for a chance to cast judgment on you. Even if you are on great terms with everybody around you, there are far too many people who would use this against you for a million different reasons. You know what I'm talking about. You may know people who seem open-minded and liberal in their views, but they couldn't handle anything like this. Even some of your best friends might start talking about you at the first sign that you might have a non-standard view of marriage—they will sell you down the road. They will tell their best friends, who will tell their friends and then your spouse will know within a matter of days.

In any case, there is enormous social pressure to remain monogamous. It makes it extremely difficult to find decent people who may want to stray from their marriage. Or to find people who are even open to that idea. To bring it up to too many of your friends is almost social suicide. There is no way to discuss this reasonably without being labeled and without risking the chance that your spouse might find out.

So the real problem is this: how can you discretely find a decent partner? Drive across town to a bar? That might work once in a while, but there are downsides to that which are very familiar to most people. Where else? At work? At the mall? There aren't very many options..

However, with the rise of the internet, there are some new and remarkable approaches to this problem. That's right, we're in a new age and the enormous power and flexibility of the internet is being used in some very innovative ways. Every time that I think that I've seen all that the internet has to offer, someone comes up with something that simply astonishes me.

But back to infidelity.

There is one website in particular which solves almost all of the usual problems. It emphasizes discretion so that you're not going to get caught. There's enough information about the other members so that you can find people who you might be interested in. And it allows you to exchange private e-mails, instant messages and phone calls so that you can get a pretty good idea of what that other person is like. There is plenty of sensible information on how to stay safe—what works and what doesn't. Do you have a pen out and are you ready to copy down this website? Well, maybe you shouldn't…just commit this memory so there's no evidence:

It's www.AshleyMadison.com.

This is your first homework assignment. The next time you're home by yourself, and fairly certain that you won't be interrupted: go check it out.

So suppose you take a look at it…what's the first thing that you'll see? Without even joining, you can get a count of how many members there are in your area. These are people who are actively cheating on their spouses. They are running around in a world that, five minutes ago, was probably unimaginable to you.

After you start to breathe again, it will take you a few minutes to join and get a free membership. At that point, you are off to the races. You can find out more about these mysterious people: you can see their pictures and read about their deepest sexual desires. Be forewarned: after the first visit, you may become a little bit obsessed. You may think about it constantly and you may be unable to focus on anything for a few days. That's normal, there are parts of your brain that are being excited that have been dead for years.

From there, you can decide how you want to use the site. Everybody is different and there are many approaches. However, there is one thing that you will notice right away.

The most popular people are the most attractive people and these people tend to be in certain weight ranges. This is important: there is pressure in this group to be slender and fit. If you are, you will get attention from some stunning people. If you are not, you may be a little disappointed with what happens. That's okay though, remember what I wrote earlier? You have the rest of your life to figure this out. You have 365 more days of losing weight before this time next year and you're going to look a million percent better.

Can you feel it yet? Do you understand this motivation? This is a sure way to lose weight. Up until now, your motivation probably came and went. For most of the day you were a true believer in sticking to your diet and exercising like a maniac. But there was always that weak point in the day, right? That hour when you open every cupboard and graze on anything you can find. At that weak point in the day, you're not thinking about the diet or the exercise. You're simply filling your belly and screwing everything up.

But if you had the possibility of meeting someone, say tomorrow. Someone new...someone gorgeous and over-sexed. They've made you laugh in their e-mails; you've found a new friend. And then, you realize, that this new someone might see you naked. No—it's more than that...the new someone will *probably* see you naked.

Trust me, you will find a new level of discipline and self-control. You might start thinking to yourself...I need to lose at least five more pounds...why am I not hungrier right now? I need to add another two miles to my run.

Does this mean that you're going to become a completely different person? Maybe yes, maybe no. The way I see it, just because you are dabbling in this sort of thing, it doesn't mean that you need to jump in with both feet. You don't need to sleep with five or six different people every week. In fact, you might just flirt with someone over the internet and that might be enough for you. Or maybe you'll be looking to find those one or two special experiences. The way I see it, I don't need to eat lobster every night, but, once in a while, a little bit of lobster is incredibly delicious—*sinfully* delicious.

There is one more interesting aspect to all this. Do you know what the warning signs of infidelity are? Amazingly, one of the well-known indicators is a sudden and dramatic weight loss—some say that this is the number one tell-tale sign that there's some hanky-panky going on. So which comes first, the weight loss or the affair? Are you losing weight so you can have an affair or are you having an affair so that you can lose the weight? Not that it matters. Remember: what's most important here is to find something that will motivate you. To find something that will help you stick through this, day by day, week after week. And if that motivation brings a little spice and a little adventure into your life, so much the better.

2. Three Rules

Now that I have your complete attention, we're going to hit some of the basics of losing weight. But before starting any weight loss program, check with your doctor to make sure that it's safe to do so. Chances are, you'll be told, "It's about dang time."

This chapter is about the three rules that you need to learn first. Much of the rest of this book contains hints and suggestions that become important as you learn more and more about these basics. You'll eventually find that, as complicated as everything sounds here, it's hard to even scratch the surface of everything that affects your weight.

But, when faced with a problem this complicated, it's best is start with something simple. We can break everything down into three simple rules. Here's the first:

Rule #1: **Regular Weigh-ins.**

The first rule is that you need to weight yourself in frequently. If you ignore everything else in this book, *do not* ignore this. Please.

Why is that? Would you drive a car without a speedometer? Do you microwave food without a timer? When you stop to think about it, just about everything that's important can be measured and is measured. The same thing is true about your weight. How else can you possibly know whether your new habits are working? How else can you know if you have been making some big mistakes?

There is one unexpected aspect of frequent weigh-ins that you will learn to appreciate. You see, the more often you weight yourself, the less you'll be intimidated by the scale; the negative emotions that most people attach to weigh-ins won't be as bad. You will find that there is less drama in stepping onto the scale and that, even if you've gained five pounds, it doesn't seem like a catastrophe any more. You may even become a little callous to the entire event. And that's a good thing…is it a big deal if you drift ten miles an hour over the speed limit? No, you check that speedometer so often that you simply let off the gas and forget about it. Weigh-ins can be almost that easy.

And remember, the more often you weigh yourself, the better you will understand your body's reactions to different foods and exercises. With every weigh-in, you'll be a little smarter and you'll be able to lose weight a little more effectively; every weigh-in is a VICTORY. In fact, I usually say that to myself as I step on the scale. "Victory!" Try it.

How should you weigh yourself?

This might seem like a stupid question, but this is important. Most people weigh themselves whenever it occurs to them: at the gym after a workout, or just before bed and they happen to see the scale out of the corner of their eye, or— most often—never (except at the doctor's office).

Here's a much better idea:

Especially when you're first starting, weigh yourself *every day* and always at the *same time* of day. Does your weight change after you've eaten dinner or after you've been in the steam room? You bet. Is that the weight loss or gain that you're trying to measure? No, it's not—you should be looking for real long-term weight loss here. You don't need to worry about the three pounds of water weight that you can lose by running a few miles or the five pounds of excrement that you just left in the toilet. So don't measure it.

The best way to get at your real weight is to weigh yourself at the same point every day. For me, the best time is first thing in the morning (after I've taken my morning pee and before I've eaten breakfast). At that point, all of my daily cycles have run their course and I'm starting from about the same point I was the day before. I believe that it's more consistent that way and consistent information is more useful.

Rule #2: **Work Toward a Goal.**

You should know exactly what your short term goal is for the next week. Losing one or two pounds per week is what the experts recommend. That sounds about right to me.

Why? A pound a week is a big enough goal so that you will know whether you made it or not. If the goal is set too low, say one pound per month, then you can always fool yourself into thinking that you can catch up by losing all the weight the last week of the month—you need to keep more pressure on yourself.

And if it's set too high, you might hurt yourself or put yourself into a position where you will get discouraged and binge. This will lead to failure. Instead, this goal needs to be small enough to be manageable.

Also, it's important to track weight from week to week. We all have different weekly habits…a weight on a Monday morning may not mean the same thing as a weight on a Friday morning. For women, there are some monthly changes that you will also begin to understand in more detail. Don't worry about those yet…the more you weight yourself, the better you will understand all these cycles.

How do I determine my goal?

You can find your ideal weight from the chart on the next page or use some other method to your liking. The weights shown here are recommendations for what an ideal weight might be for different heights. These are actually the maximum weights for large-frame people so your goal weight is likely a few pounds below these suggestions. Or, if you're interested in another method, you can use the Body Mass Index calculation (which is preferred by many experts) and there are several other ways to calculate your goal weight. There is quite a bit of discussion on which is the best method, but, don't worry too much about all that, they're all about the same. The important thing is to know what your ideal weight is. This is the weight that you're working toward. This is what you will weigh soon. That ideal weight is important…have it burned into your mind. Think about it every day.

Height	Max Weight (Women)	Max Weight (Men)
5' 2"	137 lbs	142 lbs
5' 4"	144	148
5' 6"	152	155
5' 8"	160	163
5' 10"	167	171
6'	173	179

Once you understand what your ideal weight should be, it's time to set up some short-term steps to get there. These will be your short-term goals. Every week, you're going to be a little bit closer to your ideal weight. So, how do you start?

First, write down the number after this Friday's weigh-in. Find a calendar and write down numbers every Friday. This will give you an idea of what you need to accomplish over the next weeks and months. Next Friday's goal will be this week's weight minus two pounds. If you're 160 this week, next Friday you should be at 158 and then 156 the week after. And so on until the number equals your goal weight.

As the weeks go by, write down your actual weight next to your goal weights.

At the end of each week, if you've lost two or more pounds, you can congratulate yourself—you're doing well. Keep doing exactly what you've done over the past week.

If you've lost only one, that's still okay. Try to do better.

And there's a third possibility—it's the one we don't want to think about. If you haven't lost anything or if you have gained back a little bit, you should try your best to figure out what your most serious mistakes were doing the course of the week. Remember those mistakes and do your best to avoid repeating them.

Rule #3: **Stay on the Attack**.

The third basic rule is all about how you handle your feelings about all this. Most people get nervous when a weight loss program is described as a 'life-style change' or they're lectured that this program must be followed for the 'rest of your life'. It sounds like an endless struggle. Who the hell wants to eat broccoli and run marathons every day until you die?

So they believe that they've been asked to simultaneously commit to two different types of struggles: (a) there's the physical aspect of unpleasant workouts and (b) there's the unpleasantness of the foul-tasting diet foods. And nobody really discusses the third difficulty: the emotional struggle…how can I stick with something like this for years when I can't stick to it for two days straight? I must be weak…

While it's true that this is a life-long effort, you'll soon see that it doesn't have to be a struggle. The whole approach is to pick exercises and diets that you can live with. Don't worry, with a little thought and determination, you will find a way. Then, once you've discovered a reasonable path to weight loss, you'll become more and more confident in your new mastery of your body. These things will become habits that you won't need to think about or worry about. It will no longer be a struggle. It's only a struggle if you don't understand how to lose weight. If you understand those things, then every day for 'the rest of your life' becomes an *opportunity* to lose weight. Every day is a new day to improve your body and your health. And every day you will get smarter about how to do it and you will become more confident.

As you get smarter, you will find the exercises and foods that are right for you. What are the 'right' exercises and foods? They are simply the exercises and foods that you like. Not everybody can go on a carb-free diet and not everybody can run five miles at a time. Extreme programs will work for a little while, but you're not going to stick with them, right? So, at it's core, this is really the start of a long experiment to find the foods and exercises that you're comfortable with. After all, you're just another walking-around biology experiment like me. And the two of us are a couple of experiments that should not be allowed to be out of control.

Hopefully, you're beginning to see a glimmer of hope now. And, you may not believe this yet, but this is more than just hope…this is certainty. You *will* be losing that weight and it's because you're going to be able to *stay on the attack*. You are simply going to find the easiest way to do it. There won't be any reason to backslide any more. It will all be under your control. You'll find that, once you're <u>able</u> to stay on the attack, you will be <u>eager</u> to stay on the attack.

3. More Exercising

Eat less, exercise more. You've heard that a million times by now. But every time you start an exercise program, it never seems to go anywhere. And we've all seen it: the exercise rooms are packed the first week of every January with people who are determined to follow through on New Year's resolutions. They've promised themselves that they will start a good exercise program. And every year, those same exercise rooms are nearly empty by the first week in February. Why is that? We laugh about it, but there is something real going on there. It will happen again next year and the year after. People will talk earnestly about how important it is and they will mean it. Yet, the actual exercising only lasts for about a week.

Is there something that ruins all those budding exercise programs? There must be. It's such a predictable pattern that it's obvious that, for some reason or reasons, it is very difficult to get an exercise program off the ground. Actually, I think that there are numerous things that kill exercise programs and that, with some thought, you can avoid those pitfalls.

There are five aspects to this approach:

(1) Picking your exercise.

(2) Making exercise your highest priority.

(3) Measuring your exercise.

(4) Increasing your exercise.

(5) What your exercise program should feel like.

Picking your exercise.

Obviously, there are many books, videos and TV shows that can help you with exercise. You can play sports or you can take an aerobic class. There are so many choices. What should you do?

This is simple.

Pick the ones that you enjoy (but pick several). If you don't like to run, don't. If you like riding bikes, do it. But there are other things to consider too. Is the gym too hot or cold for you? Do you have to drive too far? Are the people in that gym too creepy?

Are there ways to improve the experience? If you like music, maybe bring a CD or an MP3 player with you. If you like to read, bring a book (such as this one), or take your cell phone with you and text all your friends.

This may all seem trivial and self-absorbed, but it's not. Remember: you are setting yourself up for a long-term exercise program. Many people think of exercise in terms of how many minutes and hours they've put in lately. But that's not how it works—it has taken you months and years to put on that weight, it's going to take you months and years to lose it. So you're going to have to set up a program that you can stay with for months and years.

Make it fun. Make it so that you *want* to go get your exercise. Please understand, there will be days when it won't seem like any fun at all and you'll have to drag yourself to the gym. It happens to everybody. But, if you have the best possible plan, you might—you just might—be able to keep going.

And that's critical. Because, once you stop for a little while, it becomes difficult to get going again. So it's vital to keep going with your exercise program…even through minor injuries, bad weather, and any other difficulty you might encounter.

Making exercise your highest priority.

There are many ideas on how often and how long to exercise. Basically, you should do as much as possible without hurting yourself. If you haven't exercised in a while, you won't be very smart about what this means. So at first, it's most important to set aside some time and do something several times a week. In time, you will learn what your capabilities are.

It's also seems to be important to mix in some aerobics with some anaerobic exercises. And remember to stagger the different types of exercises so you're not doing the same thing day after day. You don't want to injure yourself and you don't want to be bored.

Here's my schedule: I exercise six times a week and take a day off to recover. I run on Tuesdays, Thursdays and Saturdays. If the weather doesn't cooperate with running, I use an exercise machine in my basement. On Mondays, Wednesdays, and Fridays; I lift weights and ride a stationary bike. My MP3 player always has some rock and roll on it that I love (for the running and the bike) and I always carry a clean set of gym clothes in my car. Do you see what I've set up? My schedule includes (1) stuff I like to do, (2) some music that I look forward to, (3) it's convenient, and (4) it's varied.

This is a schedule that I can keep.

But wait, isn't my family my highest priority? Or isn't my job my highest priority? Yes, they are. But exercise also needs to be your highest priority. Are you ever late for work? Well then, why is it acceptable to be late for your daily exercise? Would you ever think about canceling a dinner with your family? How then can you cancel a workout? See how this works? These are all your highest priorities.

And you might have to use some smarts to keep exercise as a priority. Put it on your calendar and when someone asks you to go to that movie, the answer becomes, "No, I have something else planned." Too often exercise is the lowest priority and it gets wiped out by almost anything that comes along. The time you have exercising is precious and it needs to be protected.

Measuring your exercise.

How many miles did you run? How many minutes did you use the stepper? How much weight did you bench press and how many reps did you do? How many sit-ups? How long were you peddling away on the stationary bike and at what level? You'll soon see that 10 minutes on the stationary bike will not have much of an effect on your weight loss and that you will need to stay on it for 30 or 40 minutes. In fact, there may be many things that you do that won't have an immediate effect—or even a desirable long-term effect, but that's what you want to know, isn't it? You're getting much more than just weight loss from these exercises…you'll be slowly gaining knowledge about what your body can do and how it responds. As soon as you start measuring your workout, you are much closer to understanding exactly how your body reacts to an exercise program.

And your body may react in unexpected ways. For example, I now know quite a bit about one exercise that I need in order to *maintain* my weight, I know that I need to run about five miles a few times a week. But to *lose* weight, I need to run seven to eight miles. At one point, I thought that if seven or eight miles was good, maybe running ten miles would be even better. I was sure that the weight would come off even faster if I did that. However, I soon found out that if I ran ten miles regularly, two bad things happened: (1) I tended to over-eat in an effort to replace what had been lost in the workout and, by overdoing it, it meant that I might actually gain some weight. (2) My knees and ankles couldn't take the extra mileage and I soon had trouble walking. At that point, the aches and the pains made it even more difficult to keep going with my other exercises…the entire weight loss program was in trouble.

But that's *my* body talking. It took me several years to figure out all that. So don't expect to learn everything in the first day or in the first week or even in the first month. Yet, on the very first day you will begin to learn a few things about how your body reacts to exercise. You may find out that you can't yet stay on an elliptical trainer for more than ten minutes. Does this make you a horrible person? Of course not, it just means that when your body is in an untrained state, that you should start off with a ten minute workout on the elliptical. Ten minutes—it's not very good but at least it's a start. And next week, maybe you'll see that you can increase that time to 20 or 25 minutes…then you'll have a better idea of how quickly your fitness can progress. As time goes on, you will understand more and more to the point where you will be fine-tuning your exercise schedule until it is perfected. And, after a few months of polishing your program, you will be fine-tuning it without even thinking about.

Increasing your exercise.

It happens to everybody. First you start an exercise program, then you build up your weight training and your aerobic training to what you know is a rigorous workout. Then you keep it right there for six months or longer. The body begins to adapt to that program and you might even start to slowly gain a few pounds back. At that point, you've reached a plateau and you need something to get you past it.

If you're not raising your heart rate or sweating a little bit during your workout, you might be wasting your time. If you suspect that your body is getting used to your program (and it will), try exercising a little harder or a little longer. Buy a heart rate monitor and learn how to use it.

If you're lifting weights, don't do a hundred reps with ten pounds—that's not doing anything but making some clanking noises that annoy the other people in the gym. Make sure you're completing a typical program…maybe ten reps where that tenth is making you strain. You should be slowly adding enough weight to make that last rep difficult. Or you can try different exercises. Even something as simple as adjusting your hands on the lat pull-down machine can turn it into a different exercise and it will again be a challenge.

At some point you will likely become injured or sick. After you have recovered, you cannot jump back into your exercise program where you left it. You will need to take it easy for a few sessions, maybe a week or so. Listen to your body and be careful not to re-injure yourself by getting back into your routine too quickly.

One word of caution here: when you're thinking about increasing your exercise program, try to limit your expectation of what your body can look like. There are many commercials on TV selling a wide variety of different exercise products…and they all use extremely good-looking and fit-looking people. Please note that many of those people are 'fitness models' which means they spend eight or more hours in the gym, lock themselves into diets that monks wouldn't live on, and many of them are heavy users of anabolic steroids. Those body types are not the goal and you will very likely hurt yourself by trying to increase your workout routine to look like one of those 'fitness models'.

What your exercise program should feel like.

This is critical. Every night when you go to bed, there are only two possibilities. Either you have exercised enough that day or you haven't.

If you can't tell that you've exercised during the day (and you did), then your exercise program is not yet up to speed. If you're pulling muscles and can barely walk—if you use the word 'pain' more than 'tired', then you need to throttle back a little bit on your exercise program. Here are some other descriptive words to tell if you're exercising too much: 'sore' is good, 'cramps' is not. Feeling a little tired when you're climbing up the stairs is okay, but having a pronounced limp is not. Listen to your body—being fatigued is what you want, but try not to hurt yourself. If you hurt yourself, that will only delay your weight loss program. Injuries are something that will happen in many exercise programs, but they are something to be avoided as much as possible.

Summary.

So, have you met that special someone yet? Do you think that he or she would be more attracted to you if you were in better shape? You bet they would. Or maybe you've been rejected by a few people and you're feeling discouraged by your appearance. Please don't be. You are on the right track and it won't be long before you will be in high demand. Because you now know how to start an exercise program and keep it going. And you know how to make it work, too.

This is a process. Get into a routine, but don't be afraid to change that routine. If something is easy and convenient for you, and it seems to be helping you lose weight: stick with it and try to build on it.

This is going take longer than you'd like it to and the

results will come slower than you think they should. You're not going to succeed in the next week or two. It also means that you're not going to fail either. There is always another day and another chance to learn from your mistakes.

Be careful and make slow deliberate changes to your routine. Pushing too hard will either make you miserable or injured. Either way, it's a recipe for disaster. It's a chance to quit. And you must never-never-*never* quit.

4. Less Eating

So you need to lose ten pounds. No sweets, no carbs, and no fatty foods for three months—the weight will just fall off, right? Who can't do that?

Hah!

As you may already know, that sort of plan might work for an afternoon or even a day or two, but eventually your body will have its way. You will begin to feel a little bit hungry, that hunger will steadily grow until you feel desperately hungry, and finally you will become uncontrollably hungry. *Crazy* hungry! Nothing is safe in your refrigerator or your cupboard. You might eat a huge bowl of ice cream smothered in chocolate and follow that with some potato chips. At that point, you're off the diet and, many times, you're right back into your bad old habits. All is lost.

There is a law of physics that says, "For every action, there is an equal and opposite reaction." That law seems to works for starvation diets too. Many times, a dieter is able to suffer through a difficult diet for a very long time only to lose control for a few minutes and gain all of the weight back. And maybe even gain back a little bit more.

It's heartbreaking.

It's infuriating.

But it's only natural.

However, there is hope. That hope lies in learning just how far you can push your hunger. I think of it as a zone—a weight loss zone—that is somewhere between eating too much and too little. It's a question of finding the right balance...of knowing what you're eating and making intelligent adjustments as you go. It's a matter of pacing yourself. This is one of the real secrets to true weight loss. Rejoice thee of little faith! For there is a way and you too can do it.

It's also very important to be exercising, as we discussed in the last chapter, but it's just as important to find the right diet—one that you can live with which puts you squarely into that weight loss zone. And, as before, there are five aspects to getting into the zone:

(1) Decreasing calories.
(2) Eliminating your 'disaster' foods.
(3) Identifying the foods that help.
(4) Learning to say 'No'.
(5) Managing hunger.

Decreasing calories.

It's a math problem. If you take in X number of calories, with your metabolism and your level of exercise, you will gain or lose Y number of pounds. There's nothing magical or vindictive about this. It's math. And it's a math problem that your body computes every second of every day and it never makes a computational error. So the first thing to do is to understand how many calories you're taking in. There are many calorie counters out there and calories are posted on most food packages.

Read them. Know those numbers.

You might be surprised to find out what you've been eating. Me? I was surprised as hell to find out that some delicious bread that I was using to make sandwiches had as many calories as a piece of cheesecake. It took me 20 minutes of sweating on an exercise bike to counteract the calories from just two slices of bread. Needless to say, I switched to another type of bread.

Maybe bread is not your weakness. Maybe it's something else. But the key is information. Know how many calories you are putting in your mouth.

And do not fool yourself into thinking that those 'lite' chips are only a few calories apiece. If you eat the entire bag, you need to understand how many calories are in the entire bag.

Another hint...this one is simple and direct and obvious. Please take it to heart: <u>do not eat seconds</u>. Again, this is math. When you take seconds, you are doubling your caloric intake. And, if you are doubling your caloric intake, you are going to have trouble losing weight.

Eliminating your 'disaster' foods.

For me (and for most dieters) there are a few things that ruin everything. Here are my nominations: French fries, pizza, and tortilla chips. I'm sure that you can come up with your own list of five or more diet disasters. The idea here is this: stop eating these things and you will find something better (almost anything will be better). If you don't think these things will kill your diet, count the calories.

Identifying the foods that help.

But this doesn't have to be all negative. You should be actively looking for foods that you like that help you cut down on calories. I have my secrets that may or may not work for you. Here's what I look for: a breakfast bar for breakfast, a bowl of soup for lunch, and something reasonable for dinner with some diet ice cream for desert. I even have a few cookies after dinner too. Those miniature carrots can be a great filler for me in between meals. If I really need a snack, I try to stick to nuts. Yeah sure, they're not exactly a diet food, but a handful of peanuts can quickly take care of any sort of between-meal hunger that might crop up. Find the fruits that you like and keep some around. Some crackers with a can of diet soda can also take the edge off. Of course, this all works for me…what will work for you? That's really a question that only you can answer.

Learning to say 'No'.

Often we eat out of politeness. Here's how this happens: someone brings a box of donuts to a meeting and passes it around. Or there's a birthday party and you're given the corner piece, the one with the thickest coat of frosting. The holidays are the worst time: what happens when your mom comes by with a huge piece of pumpkin pie slathered in whipped cream? It seems hopeless, doesn't it? And there will be times when you are going to lose these little games.

Even so, there may be a few tricks that you can learn that might help. Think about it, what is this really about? These little events are about relationships...family relationships, work relationships, etc, etc, etc. And when you turn down something (that you really don't want to turn down), you feel as though you're telling Cousin Marge that her Baked Alaska sucks...and, by extension, that she's a terrible cook and you don't really like her. Or you're telling your co-worker, who just turned forty-five, that he's just not that important to you—you're not interested in his birthday party. Come on! Join in! Have a little cake! It's calorie-free. Ha-ha-ha. Very funny!

It's all so ridiculous, but it's not very easy to avoid. Yet, there are some things that you can do—you can give yourself a better chance with some planning. If there is a cake in the room, go to the other side of the room. Maybe they won't chase you all the way over there. Or offer to cut your own piece...it's okay to have something if you're hungry, but make it a small one.

Another strategy is to lie. Yes, that's right. Lie. Say something that will deflect the offers. Here are a few of mine: "This is the only time of day that I have any will power, so I have to use it", or "I already had a piece". These are little white lies that will probably get you out of 90% of these situations.

And you can probably come up with some that will work for you. It takes a little preparation and a little backbone, but it is possible.

There is one lie, the big lie, that can get you out of almost any situation. Use it sparingly—it's even been known to work at family reunions and other high-risk events. "I'm feeling a little sick to my stomach. Which way is the bathroom?" That last one is particularly effective if the giver of the calories happens to be dining near you.

Managing hunger.

This is the whole point of restricting your calories. You want to feel hungry. If you're eating too much, you will not feel hungry. If you're not eating enough, you will start to feel weak and will need to binge.

First, you will need to convince yourself that it's not the end of the world if you feel a little hungry. The trick is to understand how to keep it in balance, how to keep it under control.

They say that the Eskimos have dozens of words for

snow. You should have just as many words for hunger. Let's start with the worst ...the total absence of hunger—that feeling that you get just after Thanksgiving dinner. You're bloated and maybe a little ill. You've eaten far too much and deeply regret taking that last plate of turkey. It might be hours before the tightness in your stomach goes away. This is the complete lack of hunger. This is the feeling that you never want if you're trying to lose weight.

On the other extreme, what happens if you're flying coast-to-coast on a six-hour flight, you missed breakfast and they've only fed you a small package of dry pretzels. Then there's weather at your destination and your plane has to circle for an hour and a half. At some point, the little twinge of hunger will become uncontrollable. As soon as you get into the terminal, you'll head right over to the pizza stand and get the deluxe extra-large. This is not good.

Or here's another scenario: you've just weighed in and your weight is six pounds higher than you expected. Your pants feel a little tight and you're angry with yourself. Very angry. It's taken you three months to lose that weight and in a matter of hours, you've gained it all back. So you skip breakfast, and you skip lunch. At 2, you're feeling good. You're a little hungry and you decide to keep pushing. Maybe the weight will go away as fast as it came back. Supper isn't until six and by five o'clock you're ready to eat the kibble out of the dog's dish. Maybe a handful of peanuts will help...no that didn't do the trick...maybe another handful. Then your hunger gets worse and you rip into the bag of caramel corn. By the time supper arrives, you've already eaten too many calories and you're ready to keep eating. See how it can happen? Does this sound familiar?

Well, there is a middle ground and that's the place to be. The trick is recognizing where that middle ground is.

Your goal is this: you should feel a little bit hungry for an hour or maybe two every day. If you don't feel hungry, don't eat. If everything is working right, you should have a nice healthy appetite when meal-time rolls around.

How do you know if you're hungry enough? I have a "hardtack" test. If I'm hungry enough so that hardtack tastes good, I'm on the right track. If it tastes like cardboard (as it usually does), I'm not quite hungry enough yet.

Another aspect to hunger is duration. How long can you or should you be hungry? Everybody has different limits and it's important that you learn what your safe limits are. Should you head to the refrigerator the moment you start to feel hungry? No. Should you wait for six hours before trying to curb your hunger? No. The answer is somewhere in between. The answer is learning to time your hunger to your meals. This will take practice and some experimentation.

With practice, you will gain confidence in your ability to

withstand being hungry for a little while. With practice you will be able to stay hungry for longer periods of time. And the weight can come off more quickly.

It is also crucial to avoid binging. At some point, you'll become too hungry to stand it any more and you'll feel the need to eat every fatty thing within reach—anything to make that hunger go away. My trick to avoid this is to eat a granola bar and drink some water or soda. The hunger won't stop right away, but in 15-20 minutes it will be tolerable again. And you've hopefully avoided a disaster.

Distractions can also be a big help. When you're sitting at your desk or in front of the TV it's very easy to start to thinking about how hungry you are, about how a few more calories won't hurt anything. Before you know it, you're rummaging through the kitchen looking for anything that will fit in your mouth, right? It doesn't have to be like that. A simple way to avoid this pitfall is to find something distracting to do which doesn't give you the opportunity to eat. Exercise can do it. If you know that you're susceptible to binging just before suppertime (like me), then that's a great time to schedule your run. Of if you have a habit of eating too much dark chocolate about an hour after supper, that might be a good time to go to the mall and do a little shopping. Just pick a mall that doesn't sell the kind of chocolate that you like.

Here's something else to think about…it's okay to be ever-so-slightly hungry at the end of the meal. Really, it is! You're not going to die or faint from lack of calories. It takes a little while for your appetite to go away after you've eaten so give your body a chance to tell you that it's full.

Overall, there is a daily food cycle to your body and it's important that you get to know it. For me, it begins as I'm going to sleep at night. At this point, I like to be ever so slightly hungry. That means that I will wake up with a nice healthy appetite. I have a small breakfast and head off to work. At work, I'm distracted from hunger until about noon. I usually get in a little exercise around lunchtime and eat a light lunch.

By late in the afternoon, I'm ready for supper. This is the most dangerous time for me…this is when I can 'make it or break it'. During supper, I do not get seconds and I do not load up my plate, especially with high calorie foods.

Sometimes—especially after a good session in the gym—I can get a little too hungry at night. This is a good time for a small snack…maybe some low fat jerky or some nuts. Eating these foods can also be tricky (at least for me). It's very easy to tell yourself that you need an extra handful of peanuts or you're going to be too hungry later.

I think of this as the second 'make it or break it' point in the day. And you're going to face points like that every day.

Sometimes eating a little bit is the right thing to do; sometimes it's not. Sometimes you'll make the right decision; other days you won't.

And, rest assured, you will make mistakes. But try to learn from them and improve. Every day you will be smarter than the last. Every day you will get better at controlling your diet.

One added bonus: every minute that you feel hungry will make it that much easier the next day. I'm convinced that we all need to build up a tolerance to feeling hungry (up to a point). So at first, it will seem very unnatural and somewhat unpleasant, but before too long, you'll expect to hear your stomach rumbling once in a while. It just takes a little getting used to.

Summary.

Diets are about balance. Not too much and not too little. The trick is finding that area that is just right. A little uncomfortable but not intolerable. That's what it's all about.

You're going to feel a little bit hungry at times. You're going to have to tell yourself that it's okay to feel a little bit hungry. And you're going to learn when it's time to head off a binge. But you'll want to do it. You need to do it. Did you see the picture that person just sent you by e-mail? It was gorgeous! How could someone like that be interested in you? Well, if those next ten pounds come off quickly enough, maybe you'll find out.

5. Understanding Your Weight

Every day you weigh-in is a victory, because every time you weigh-in you will be faced by a number. That number is almost always higher or lower than it was the day before, and you will wonder why. You can't help it—it's natural to be curious...you will try to figure out what happened.

And every time you check your weight and think about why it changed, you will learn more and more about how things affect your body.

Sometimes your weight goes up and the reason is

obvious: you've eaten too much or you haven't been able to exercise.

Sometimes your weight goes down and the reason is obvious: you've been good and you've managed to stick to your plan.

But then there are going to be the days when it's not clear what happened. Maybe you ran five miles the day before, skipped dessert, and gained three pounds despite it all. You don't remember eating all that much, but there it is, there's that number and it might even make you a little angry. The scale must be lying. The scale hates you, right? It can't be right.

Well, perhaps. But it's better to think about things in terms of math. That number on the scale needs to be addressed. You might have eaten too much or you may have exercised too little.

Yet there may be other reasons for that number. Remember, this can be more complicated that you might think. So before you get too excited about a little weight gain, let's talk about a few possibilities...

Bowel movements...this is a little gross, but this might be the culprit. If you haven't gone in a day or two, you may be carrying around an extra pound or two. Or, if you've had diarrhea, you might be a little lighter.

Water weight: there are many factors that can affect this.

Hard workouts and long plane rides tend to dehydrate me and I will weigh less than I expect. Or if I drink a few too many cans of diet soda, I can add a pound or even two…I suspect that I get a little bloated because of some of the chemicals in the soda. All this can add or subtract several pounds for no apparent reason. I even suspect that the humidity in the air can affect weight. I swear that on dry days I weigh two to three pounds less than on days when the humidity is high or when it's raining.

There are other factors too. Does stress affect your body? Of course it does! What if you have to concentrate on something important for several hours straight? Something like driving long distance, for example…what about that? Can that affect your weight? I think it can. For me, driving for five or six hours is almost as good as a light workout. Physically, there's not much to do, but the extra stress gets your heart rate up a little bit and boosts your metabolism. That's why you feel tired after a long drive.

Sometimes I can see a weight gain two or even three days after I've eaten too much. Why is that? I suspect that there are some foods that take a little longer to metabolize. The same thing is true if I've been good about the diet: there are times when the weight doesn't go down until a day or two later.

Now to be fair, I'll probably never get any of this

published in a professional journal (not that I'm going to try). However, I don't feel the need to prove these ideas because, after thousands of weigh-ins, it's clear to me that they're true.

And that's what you're really trying to do…you will slowly start to understand the vast complexities of what your body is going through. Can you see what is going to happen? If you have a fairly good idea of what you're putting in your body (by watching those calories), and you have a good idea of what you're taking out of your body (by measuring your exercise). Then you'll start to get a pretty good idea of how everything else affects your body.

And once you understand all that. You can make adjustments here and there and, for the first time, truly be able to lose weight. Up until now, you've only been guessing. You really didn't understand the effect that this food or that exercise had on your body. But the more you pay attention, the more you will learn and the more you will know. You will get better and better at controlling your weight. You will get more and more confident.

So you say you need to lose 10 pounds for a class reunion this summer? Or do you think that you're latest on-line 'friend' might show you a little more attention if you were 15 pounds slimmer? Or maybe you had a date at the local coffee house and the call for a second date never came.

Once, problems like that might have made you feel hopeless. You would have resigned yourself to the situation and tried something else. Maybe you would have tried dating fat people. Or flirting with that clerk at the grocery store who nobody wants to talk to.

Don't do that now. You're on the verge of being able to take control of your weight so that you can date the people you want to date. Sure, this might be a little difficult at first.. But, after you've been doing this for a few months, it won't be a problem at all.

6. Maintaining Your Weight

At some point, you will reach your goal weight.

I reached mine a few years ago and kept it. It's about ten pounds over my ideal weight, but that's okay with me. I carry a little extra muscle from lifting weights, and I feel great—my blood pressure is good and my cholesterol levels are healthy. My doctor even agrees that this is a good weight for me. This feels about right to me.

So let's assume that you've reached your goal weight too. Now comes another tricky part—the really difficult part.

You may be surprised to hear that; you may have thought that most of the problems were behind you. Not quite...

You've spent months and months feeling a little bit hungry for a few hours at a time. At times, you probably thought of this as slow torture and you probably thought about giving up a dozen times every day. Well, the good news is that the slow torture is over.

It's time to stop that.

It's time to ease up ever so slightly, but you must be careful to stay with your exercise schedule and continue to limit your food intake.

You still need to feel a little bit hungry a few times a day.

And you still need to feel a little tired from your workouts.

Most importantly, keep weighing in. You'll probably gain back a few pounds and when that happens, it's time to start dieting again.

I feel as though any weigh-in that gives me a number that is five pounds more than my target weight warrants a new diet. But who cares? You know exactly how to lose that weight, just apply yourself and your accumulated knowledge and that five pounds will be gone before you know it. A small increase like that is not a big deal.

However—beware. There are some real dangers once you try to 'level off' at your goal weight. This is the time when it's very easy to revert to your old habits. These are the habits that will add all the lost weight back and maybe even add a few more pounds on top of it all. And when you add back that much weight, it is a big deal.

And sadly, *you will probably add that weight back.*

At least once or twice.

That's what the statistics tell us. It happens to almost everybody. Even the people who have lost a significant amount of weight and eventually keep it off...they have lost and gained that weight several times before finally keeping it off for good. This might be the hardest part of all.

So now it's time for round two...

Oh now, not *Round Two!*

I know what you're thinking: that won't be me. If I ever lost 30 pounds, I would never-ever-never gain it back.

Well, I hope you're right, but I'd bet a ton of money that you're wrong. That is a terrible thing to say, I know—I know! But this is how it works. This is how your body works and this is how your mind works.

So what exactly happens?

There may be a million ways that the weight comes back, but I know what happened to me. Twice.

And, in retrospect, it happened because I didn't think

clearly about what was happening and I allowed my emotions to control important aspects of my life.

After I lost the weight, I kept up my exercise program (or so I thought), and I stuck to my diet (or so I thought).

However, I stopped weighing myself. I thought I had the whole deal mastered and I no longer needed the stress of the scale every morning. At that point, it became easy to fool myself that I was maintaining my weight. Even while I was gaining weight, I was sure that I was actually losing weight. Talk about delusions!

For example, I remember coming home after a hard workout and feeling absolutely ravenous. I'd been exercising for several hours so I was sure that I'd burned more than my share of calories. So it didn't really matter what I ate.

So I ate three quarters of a pizza.

I know, typing that I feel like an idiot. And even while I was eating it, my brain was trying to tell me that something was very wrong. However, my legs were screaming something else: "we're sore, we need nourishment, keep eating and soon we'll feel better…we'll be stronger and then we can exercise even longer and we'll be able to lose even more weight…by eating that pizza, you're really helping your diet."

Yikes!

What was really happening was that I was over-exercising and then over-compensating. And I didn't realize this because I didn't weigh myself.

Here's something else that will throw you off: vacations and business trips. I'm probably not going to say what you think I'm going to say. Most weight loss books advise you to stick to your exercise routine and your diet when you're on the road. There's nothing wrong with that. Do your best. Try to plan ahead and find a hotel with a workout room, order the low-cal meal on the plane, and bring your running shoes.

However, in the real world, things don't always happen according to plan ...the workout room is closed, the flight attendant knows nothing about the low-cal meal, and you can't run because there are no sidewalks near your hotel.

Whenever you leave your home, your program is going to be a little out of control and you're going to stray from your carefully engineered program. It's almost unavoidable.

But that's not when the real problem happens.

It happens when you get back. You're riddled with guilt about the greasy fish and chips that you ate in San Francisco...you're ashamed of the half-pound of fresh fudge that you gobbled down in a two bites on the boardwalk...that huge western omelet at the airport wasn't very good but it sure disappeared in a hurry. That's all you can remember: a week and a half of eating, eating, and more eating. Worse yet, there was absolutely no exercise to balance it out.

You're sure that you've gained ten pounds, maybe twenty. And *that's* when you make your biggest mistake...

You decide to skip the weigh-in.

For just this one time, you can't face it. It would be devastating to get on the scale and see the new number. And, you think, it went on so quickly; I can take it off just as quickly. This is just a temporary blip and in a few days I'll be back down to a reasonable weight. You'll figure that you can diet and exercise for a few days and get all that baby fat off. It went on fast; it'll come off fast. And then that number on the scale won't be so traumatic.

So you skip a day.

And another day.

Then a week goes by and you haven't weighed yourself. You can't seem to control yourself around food and you're more nervous than ever about weighing in. Then a month goes by and you've pretty much forgotten about the weigh-ins. You might even be congratulating yourself...you never needed that scale in the first place—you're looking okay in the mirror. Why stress out over a little number?

The months fly by and pretty soon your pants don't fit any more. And maybe you've split the rear end of a pair of old shorts. You've started to notice that it's not so easy to climb a flight of stairs and that you're breathing hard when you reach the top.

This has already become a disaster. This is exactly how you can gain all that weight back and more.

I know. Remember, this happened to me <u>twice</u>.

There's only one thing to do at that point: Start over.

Start the weigh-ins and the hunger hours.

Re-read this book again; you'll be surprised at how much you've forgotten (by the way, that was my initial motivation for writing this book…so that I wouldn't forget these things) and how much you've been ignoring.

Find out where your diet has failed and make sure that your exercise program is up to snuff.

You're going to be angry with yourself. Try not to be. This happens to hundreds of thousands of people. It's a trap that almost everybody falls into. It's a trap that very few people manage to escape.

This is the point where you're going to have to be very determined.

This is the point where it will take all your willpower to get going again.

What you do at this moment will determine whether you really are going to keep that weight off.

You must be strong!

The important thing is to keep trying. Keep going and get back on that scale. Even if you've gained thirty pounds, getting on that scale is a victory.

Even if you forget everything else in this book, remember this: getting on that scale is always a victory.

Getting on the scale is always the key.

7. Checklists

Initial weight loss

- ☐ I weigh-in every day.
- ☐ I weigh-in first thing in the morning.
- ☐ I write down my Friday morning weight.
- ☐ I've established my goal weight.
- ☐ I've written down my weekly goals (2 lb/week).
- ☐ I feel a little hungry for more than an hour before meals.
- ☐ I have a good exercise schedule.
- ☐ I have cut back on calories.
- ☐ I am not eating seconds at mealtime.

Maintaining my weight

- [ ] I weigh-in at least three times per week.
- [ ] I weigh-in first thing in the morning.
- [ ] My Friday morning weight isn't five pounds high.
- [ ] I feel a little hungry for an hour before meals.
- [ ] I understand why I've gained or lost weight recently.
- [ ] I keep to my exercise schedule.

Losing the weight again

- [ ] I weigh-in every day.
- [ ] I weigh-in first thing in the morning.
- [ ] I write down my Friday morning weight.
- [ ] I've written down my weekly goals (2 lbs/week).
- [ ] I feel a little hungry for more than an hour before meals.
- [ ] I have a good exercise schedule.
- [ ] I have cut back on calories.
- [ ] I am not eating seconds at mealtime.

8. A Final Thought

I truly hope that this program works for you. Nothing would make me happier than to think that I've helped even one person lose weight.

And when you're winning this battle, you might think about lending this book to a friend (but perhaps not your spouse). Tell them how it helped you learn about what works and what doesn't. But do it gently, what works for you may not work for them. They need to start learning just as you did.

The funny thing is that most people don't want to hear about diets. They have their own ideas and would rather be left alone. That's fine…I was like that once, too.

However, you need to understand one more thing. If you have dropped a significant amount of weight and have kept it off, you have joined a _very_ special club. There are very few people who have done that and many of your friends will recognize this.

You'll see it in their eyes.

No, it's not jealousy. It's a profound respect. They sense what you've done. They know that you've climbed a mountain and that you know things that they don't.

You see, most times people really don't listen to your opinions and ideas on almost anything, but this time it's different—they just might listen to you. Why is that? You're not a doctor or a dietician or an aerobics instructor.

But they'll take one look at you in your new clothes and they'll realize something: you've done it.

You've beaten the food and the exercise and the roiling months of emotion. You have controlled things that most people have no hope of controlling. In that respect, you're a better person and, inside, they want to be like you.

One look at you and they'll want know your secrets.

But before you get your friends started—before you

make them into happier and healthier people—I think you have something important to tell yourself. Go ahead, say it now—say it aloud:

I know how to lose weight!